Treatment of Lumbar Disk Herniation

Solutions for Relief Pain & Vertebral Decompression.

By Edgar Ortega M.

Edgar Ortega M.

2014 All Rights Reserved.

1st Edition

ISBN: 978-1-312-57243-0

Printed in Spain

What is Herniated Disk?

The spine is made up of a series of connected bones called "vertebrae." The disc is a combination of strong connective tissues that hold one vertebra to the next, and acts as a cushion between the vertebrae. The disc is made of a tough outer layer called the "annulus fibrosus" and a gel-like center called the "nucleus pulposus." As you get older, the center of the disc may start to lose water content, making the disc less effective as a cushion.

This may cause a displacement of the disc's center (called a herniated or ruptured disc) through a crack in the outer layer. Most disc herniations occur in the bottom two discs of the lumbar spine, at and just below the waist.

Sometimes called a slipped or ruptured disk, a herniated disk most often occurs in your lower back. It is one of the most common causes of low back pain, as well as leg pain (sciatica).

Between 60% and 80% of people will experience low back pain at some point in their lives. A high percentage of people will have low back and leg pain caused by a herniated disk.

Although a herniated disk can sometimes be very painful, most people feel much better with just a few weeks or months of non-surgical treatment.

Anatomy

Your spine is made up of 24 bones, called vertebrae, that are stacked on top of one another. These bones connect to create a canal that protects the spinal cord.

Five vertebrae make up the lower back. This area is called your lumbar spine.

Other parts of your spine include:

Spinal cord and nerves. These "electrical cables" travel through the spinal canal carrying messages between your brain and muscles.

Intervertebral disks. In between your vertebrae are flexible intervertebral disks. They act as shock absorbers when your walk or run.

Intervertebral disks are flat and round, and about a half inch thick. They are made up of two components:

- Annulus fibrosus. This is the tough, flexible outer ring of the disk.

- Nucleus pulposus. This is the soft, jelly-like center of the disk.

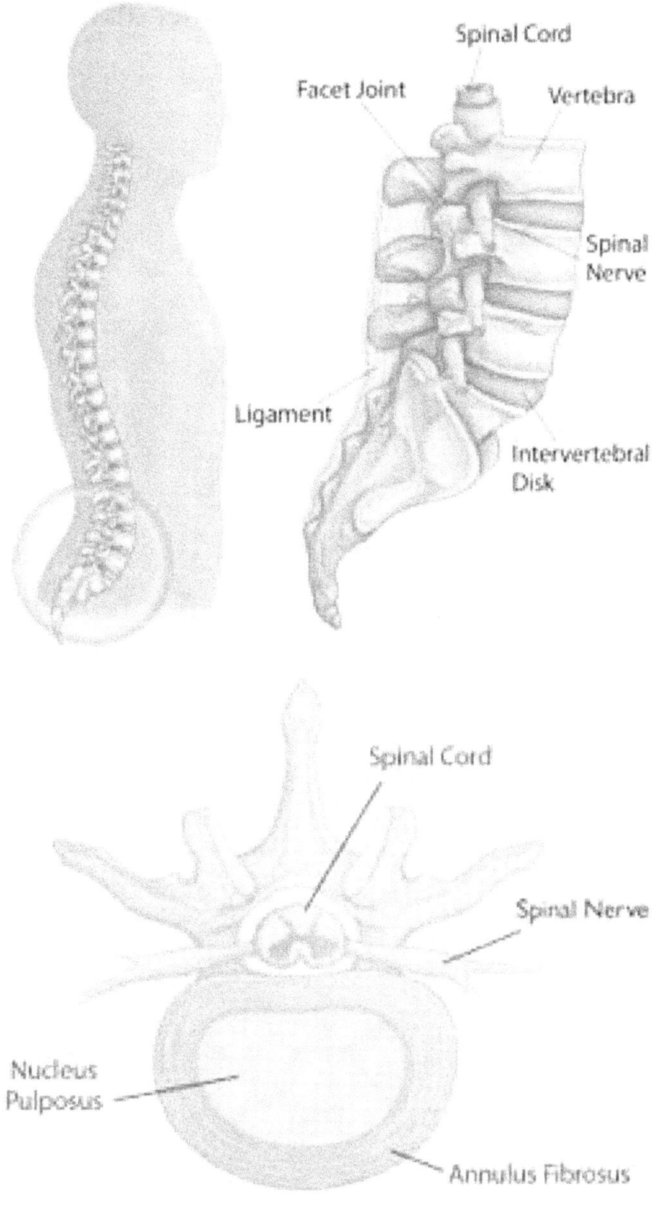

Disk Herniation

A **herniated lumbar disc** can press on the nerves in the spine and may cause pain, numbness, tingling or weakness of the leg called "sciatica."

Sciatica affects about

1-2% of all people, usually between the ages of 30 and 50.

A herniated lumbar disc may also cause back pain, although back pain alone (without leg pain) can have many causes other than a herniated disc.

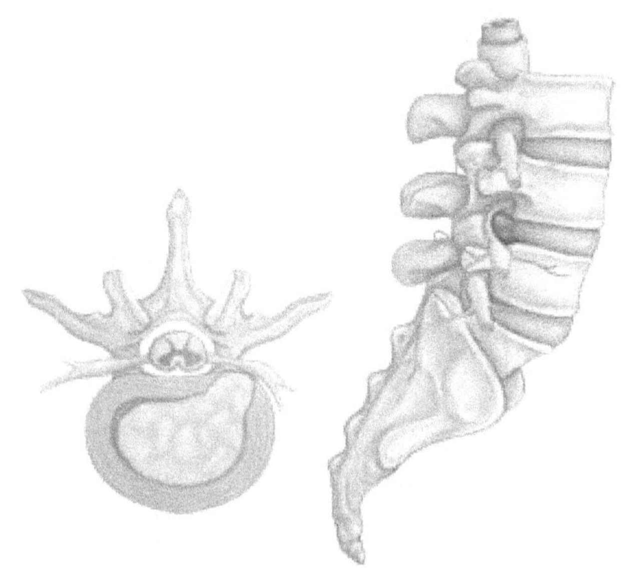

Vertebral Column Anatomy

When viewed from the side, the spine and its curves resemble a doublé S. These curves - called lordosis or kyphosis, depending on the **position ensure that the body is able to absorb impacts and leaps and is optimally supported. When viewed from behind, a healthy spine looks like a straight rod.**

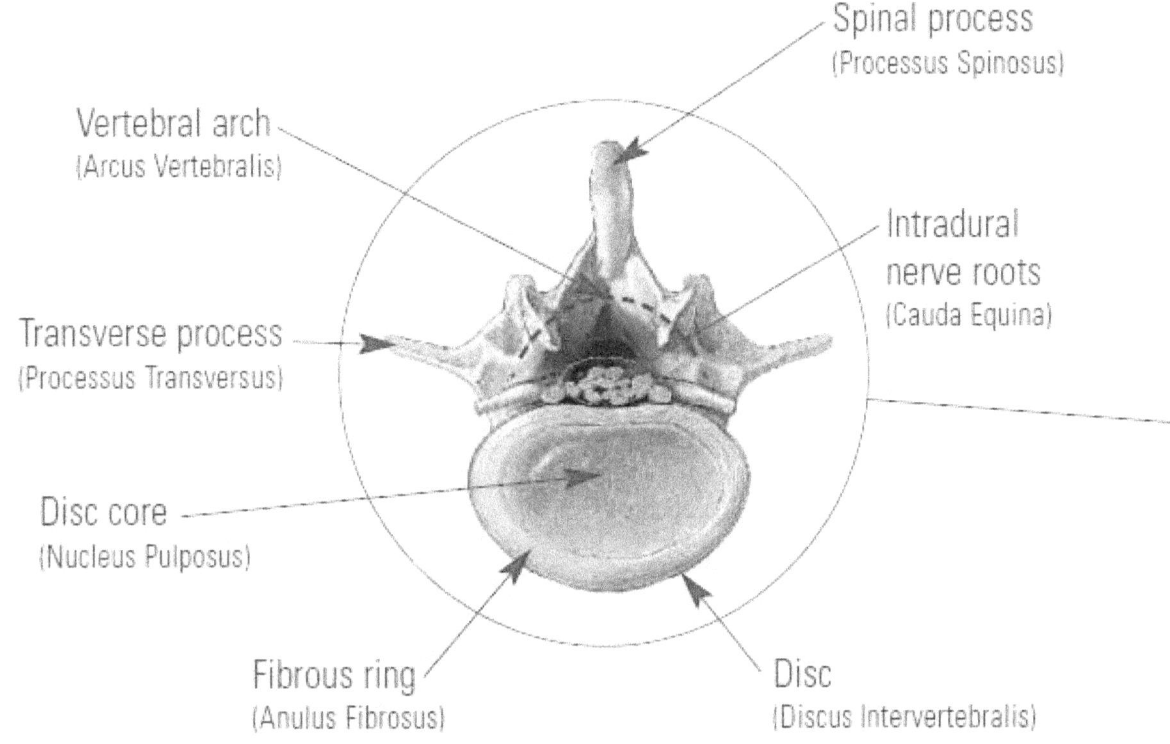

With a total of 24 vertebras, the spine is divided into three sections: the cervical spine (7 cervical vertebras), the thoracic spine (12 thoracic vertebras) and the lumbar spine (5 lumbar vertebras). The sacrum and coccyx (or tailbone), consisting of ten vertebras in total and fusing to form a bone block between the ages of 20 and 25 years, are connected to the lumbar spine.

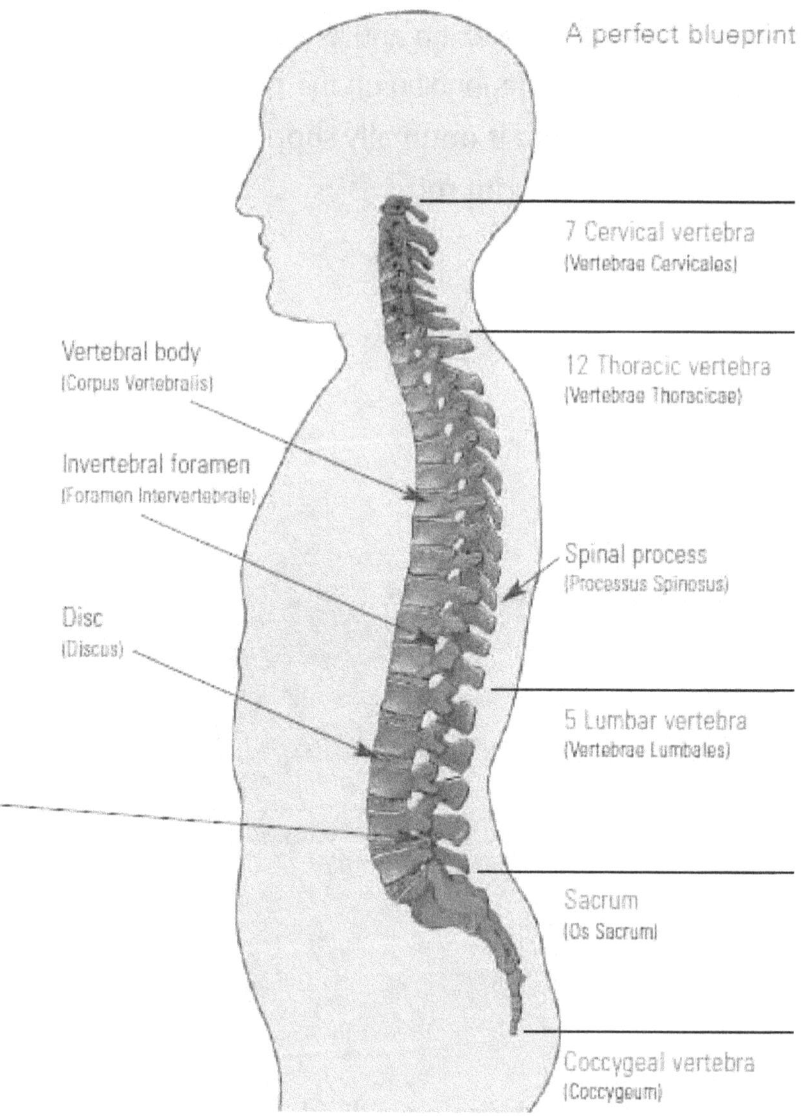

A vertebra consists of a solid frontal vertebral body and the narrower vertebral arch with vertebral joints and vertebral processes behind.

The vertebral body functions like a carrier, with the spinal marrow and intradural nerve fibers proceeding through the protected canal consisting of vertebral arches (vertebral canal and hard dura). The muscles are attached to the two transverse processes and the spinal process.

The discs act as buffers between the individual vertebrae. With their gel-like, soft, water-filled core – which is surrounded by a cartilaginous fibrous ring – they cushion any impact and allow better vertebra mobility.

An intervertebral foramen – from which the spinal nerves protrude to the left and right sides, thus leaving their protected area – is located **between the vertebra and the disc.**

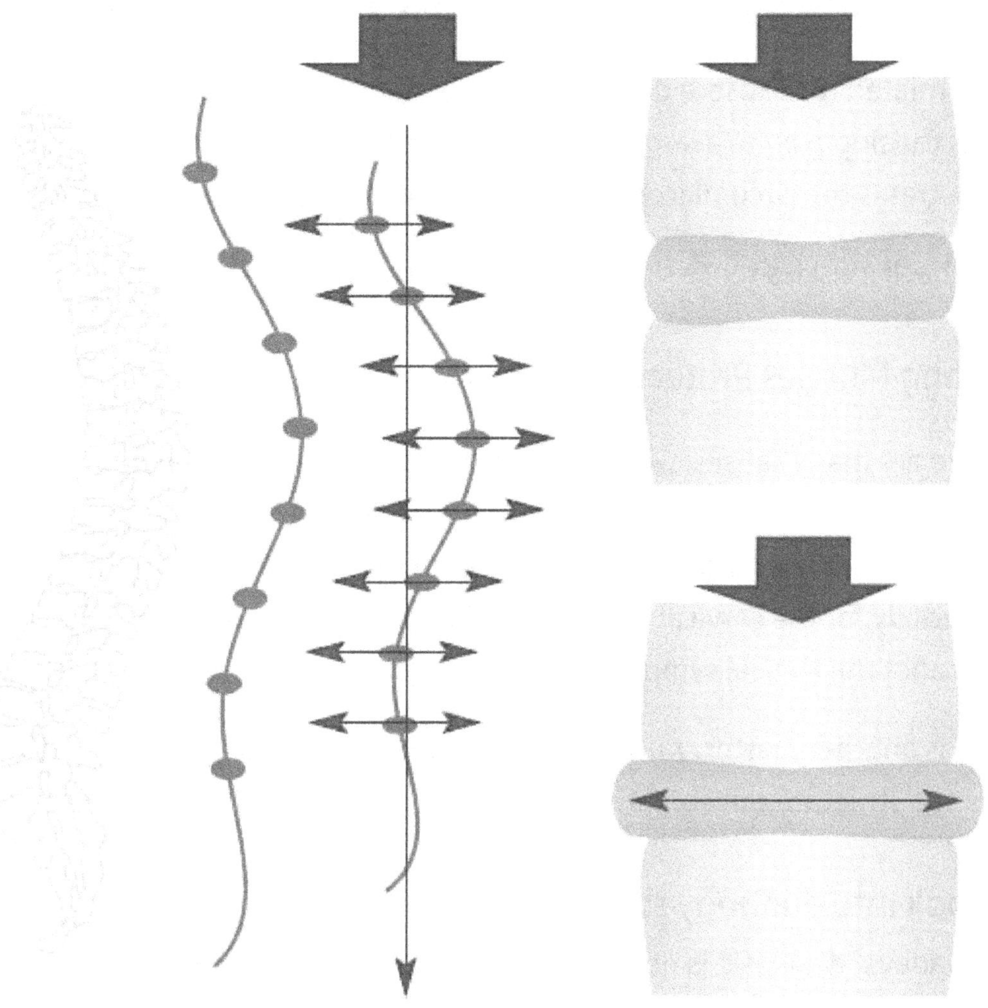

The Spine Under Pressure – The Herniated Disc

A herniated (prolapsed) disc occurs when parts of the disc slip into the vertebral canal, thus causing pain to a larger or lesser degree. The reason: the soft, gel-like disc core penetrates the circumjacent fiber jakket and presses on the surrounding nerve tissue.

The back muscles tense simultaneously, causing additional pain.

Strong Muscles Protect

There are many causes: weak stomach and back muscles, predominantly seated activities, excess weight and unfavorable body postures during everyday life (for example, using wrong lifting techniques or continuous or long driving hours, especially for the cervical spine). Hereditary malposition of the spine and pregnancies also abet the clinical symptoms.

Age is another matter, with loss of liquid from the discs increasing over the years. This porous structure can sometimes cause the disc core to leak and create a herniation.

A look into our body sheds light on the topic

Nowadays, diagnosis is generally performed with the help of MRI – magnetic resonance imaging. This gentle, non-radioactiveimaging procedure uncovers protruding or herniated discs.

A computer tomography (CT) also provides excellent results.

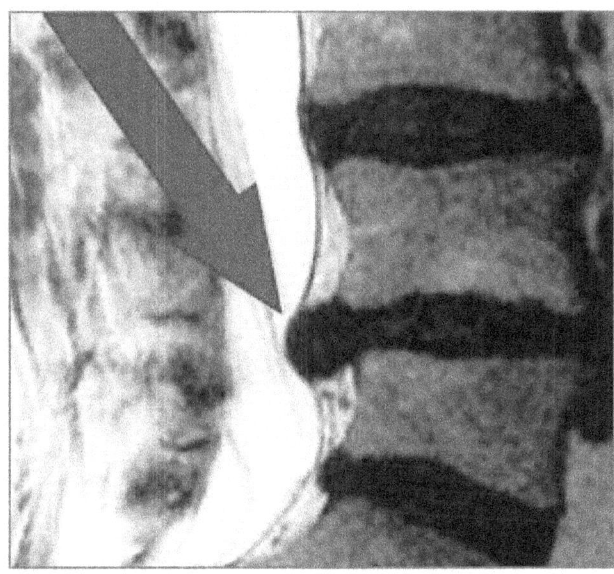

A herniated disc need not automatically cause pain. Problems especially arise when the protruding disc presses on the surrounding nerves. This often leads to severe backache, which radiates into the legs and at worst may cause a feeling of numbness, paralysis or even organic dysfunction (e.g. bladder and intestinal problems).

Such a severe herniated disc rarely comes out of the blue, even if one awkward movement may sometimes be the straw that breaks the camel's back (or yours, in this case). However, in most cases the back has already been previously affected – sometimes even without the knowledge of the person concerned.

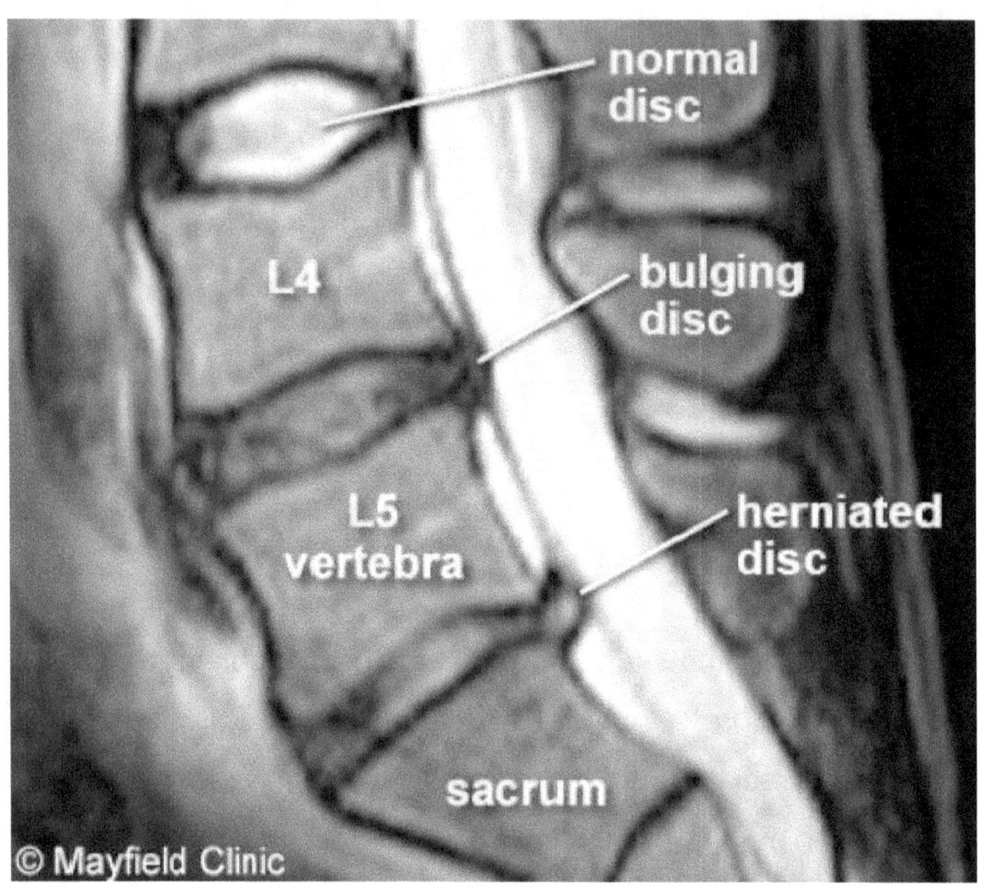

The Physical Exam

Abdomen: Palpate for pulsatile mass and tenderness

Back:

• Palpate for tenderness **midline and paraspinous**

• Percussion-induced back pain suggests spinal infection or malignancy

Straight-Leg Raise (SLR) Manuevers:

• Stretches sciatic nerve when elevate supine patient's extended leg

• Radiation of pain distal to knee suggests radiculopa**thy**

• Sensitivity = 80%, specificity = 40%

• More specific test for L5-S1 radiculopathy (sciatica) is crossed-SLR test, where pain radiates down affected

> **leg when contralateral leg is raised (sensitivity 25%, specificity 90%)**

• An L5-S1 radiculopathy is 95% **sensitive for lumbar disk herniation (thus, the absence of radiculopathy almost rules-out a herniated disk)**

• Reverse SLR: Stretches L3 and L4 nerves by elevating PRONE patient's extended leg

> **Reproduction of pain in L3-L4 distribution with reverse SLR suggests L3-L4 radiculopathy**

Neurologic:

• **Sensory:**

> **Light touch and pinprick testing of each nerve dermatome, and saddle distribution (inner proximal thighs and buttocks)**
>
> Best to perform at most distal site (foot for L4, L5, S1 – see figure below)

• **Motor: Specificity of following findings for lumbar disk herniation:**

> **Weakness of ankle dorsiflexion (70%)**
>
> **Weakness of great toe extension (70%)**
>
> **Weakness of ankle plantar flexion (95%)**
>
> **Weakness of knee extension (99%)**

• **Reflexes**

• **Gait: Spinal stenosis patients often walk with spinal flexion (bending forward)**

Rectal exam: For patients exhibiting severe back pain, bilateral leg symptoms, or

bowel/bladder changes (to check
for decreased tone, as found in cord compression and cauda equina syndrome)
Vascular:
• Check pedal pulses to help distinguish vascular claudication versus spinal stenosis
pseudoclaudication
• A decreased pulse is worrisome for acute limb ischemia (thromboembolic disease,
AAA, aortic dissection)

Waddell's signs:
• SLR exam in seated position by extending knee, should also reproduce L5-S1
radiculopathy pain
• Hyperesthesia of skin along back suggests a non-organic etiology for back pain.
• Pain with axial loading on scalp should not elicit back pain (It may, however, elicit
neck pain.)
• Over-exaggeration of pain suggests a non-organic etiology for back pain

Nerve Root Level	L3	L4	L5	S1
Pain Location	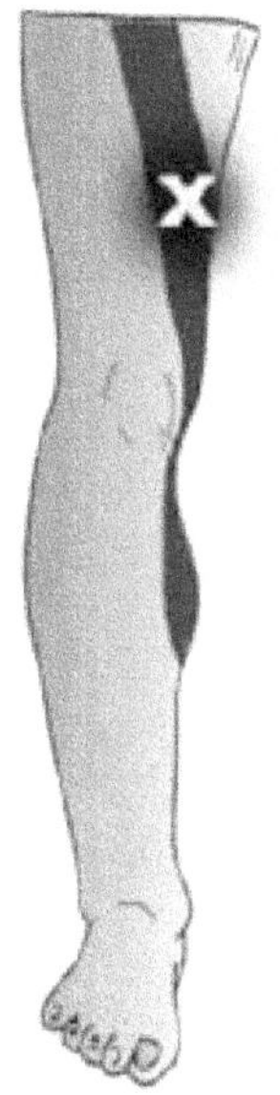	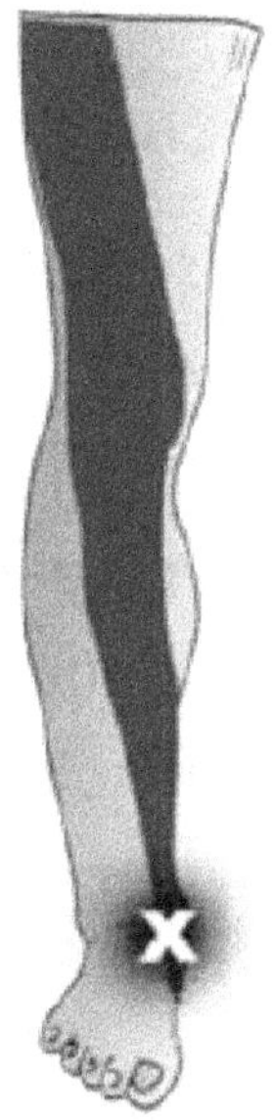	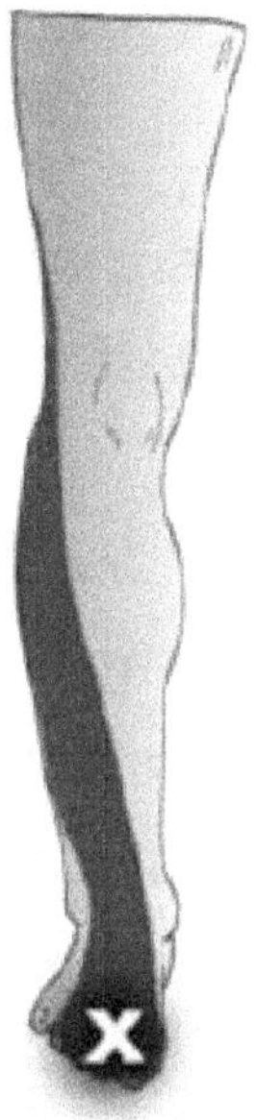	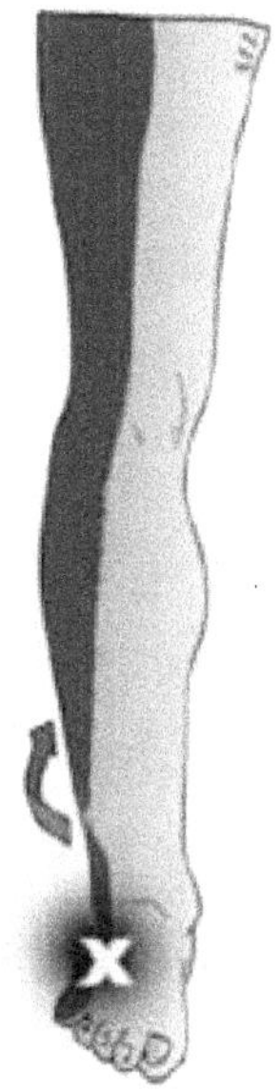
Stress Test	R-SLR	R-SLR	SLR, C-SLR	SLR, C-SLR
Sensation ("X")	Medial Thigh	Medial Foot	Between 1st-2nd Toe	Lateral Foot
Strength	Hip Flexion	Knee Extension	Big Toe / Ankle Dorsiflexion	Ankle Plantar Flexion
Reflex	---	Patellar	---	Achilles

Herniated Disk Symptoms

Herniated discs are a common source of back pain. However, symptoms alone are not enough to diagnose a herniated disc.

Your medical history is key to a proper diagnosis. A physical examination can usually determine which nerve roots are affected and how seriously. A simple x-ray may show evidence of disc or degenerative spine changes. An MRI (magnetic resonance imaging) is usually the most accurate (and most expensive) testing option to determine which disc has herniated.

Pain and other symptoms from a herniated disc can vary widely from one person to the next. Complaints range from local pain to radiating pain. Depending on where the herniation is, you may experience arm pain or leg pain in addition to back pain.

One of the most common set of symptoms associated with a herniated disc is sciatica. Contrary to popular opinion, sciatica is actually a set of symptoms and not a condition in and of itself.

When a herniated disc presses on the sciatic nerve it often leads to one or more of these symptoms:

- Sharp, shooting pain starting in the buttocks that travels down the back of one leg
- Numbness and tingling in one leg (pins & needles)
- A burning pain centered in the lower back
- Back pain with gradually increasing leg pain
- Weakness in one leg or both legs
- Loss of bladder or bowel control

While these are the most common symptoms of the condition, keep in mind that you may experience multiple symptoms from a herniated disc... or even none at all.

What are the causes?

Discs can bulge or herniate because of injury and improper lifting or can occur spontaneously. Aging plays an important role. As you get older, your discs dry out and become harder. The tough fibrous outer wall of the disc may weaken, and it may no longer be able to contain the gel-like nucleus in the center. This material may bulge or rupture through a tear in the disc wall, causing pain when it touches a nerve. Genetics, smoking, and a number of occupational and recreational activities may lead to early disc degeneration.

Who is affected?

Herniated discs are most common in people in their 30s and 40s, although middle aged and older people are slightly more at risk if they're involved in strenuous physical activity.

Lumbar disc herniation is one of the most common causes of lower back pain associated with leg pain, and occurs 15 times more often than cervical (neck) disc herniation. Disc herniation occurs 8% of the time in the cervical (neck) region and only 1 to 2% of the time in the upper-to-mid-back (thoracic) región

What treatments are available?

Conservative nonsurgical treatment is the first step to recovery and may include medication, rest, physical therapy, home exercises, hydrotherapy, epidural steroid injections (ESI), chiropractic manipulation, and pain management. With a team approach to treatment, 80% of people with back pain improve in about 6 weeks and return to normal activity. If you don't respond to conservative treatment, your doctor may recommend surgery.

Nonsurgical Treatments

Self care: In most cases, the pain from a herniated disc will get better within a couple days and completely resolve in 4 to 6 weeks. Restricting your activity, ice/heat therapy, and taking over the counter medications will help your recovery (see Self Care for Neck & Back Pain).

Medication: Your doctor may prescribe pain relievers (opioids), nonsteroidal anti-inflammatory medications (NSAIDs), muscle relaxants, and steroids.

• Nonsteroidal anti-inflammatory drugs
(NSAIDs), such as aspirin, naproxen (Alleve, Naprosyn), ibuprofen (Motrin, Nuprin, Advil), and celecoxib (Celebrex), are used to reduce inflammation and relieve pain.

• **Analgesics**, such as acetaminophen (Tylenol), can relieve pain but don't have the antiinflammatory effects of NSAIDs. Long-term use of analgesics and NSAIDs may cause stomach ulcers as well as kidney and liver problems.

In case of severe pain the opioid self administration is most common. This medications include, morphine, oxicodone, hydrocodone, buprenorphine, tramadol and codeine.

• Muscle relaxants, such as methocarbamol (Robaxin), carisoprodol (Soma) and cyclobenzaprine (Flexeril), may be prescribed to control muscle spasms.

• Steroids may be prescribed to reduce the swelling and inflammation of the nerves. They are taken orally (as a Medrol dose pack) in a tapering dosage over a five-day period. It has the advantage of providing almost immediate pain relief within a 24-hour period.

• Steroid injections into the area of your herniated disc may be prescribed if your pain is severe (see Epidural Steroid Injections). This procedure, performed under fluoroscopy, involves an injection of steroids and an analgesic-numbing agent into the epidural space of the spine to reduce the swelling and inflammation of the nerves. About 50% of patients will notice relief after an epidural injection, although the results tend to be temporary.

Repeat injections, at 2-week intervals, may be necessary to obtain the best results in the shortest time. If the injection is helpful, it can be done up to three times a year.

Physical therapy: The goal of physical therapy is to help you return to full activity as soon as possible and prevent re-injury. Physical therapists can instruct you on proper posture, lifting, and walking techniques, and they'll work with you to strengthen your lower back, leg, and stomach muscles.

They'll also encourage you to stretch and increase the flexibility of your spine and legs. Exercise and strengthening exercises are key elements to your treatment and should become part of your life-long fitness (see Physical Therapy).

Holistic therapies: Some patients want to try holistic therapies such as acupuncture, acupressure nutritional supplements, and biofeedback. The effectiveness of these treatments for a herniated disc may help you learn coping mechanisms for managing pain as well as improving your overall health.

Surgical Treatments

Surgery for a herniated lumbar disc, called a discectomy, may be an option if your symptoms do not significantly improve with conservative treatments. Surgery may also be recommended if you have signs of nerve damage, such as weakness or loss of feeling in your legs.

Microsurgical discectomy:

The surgeon makes a 1–2 inch incision in the middle of your back. To reach the damaged disc, the spinal muscles are dissected and moved aside to expose the vertebra. A portion of the bone is removed to expose the nerve root and disc.

The portion of the ruptured disc that touches your spinal nerve is carefully removed using special instruments. About 80–85% of patients successfully recover from a discectomy and are able to return to their normal job in approximately 6 weeks [2].

Minimally invasive microendoscopic discectomy:

The surgeon makes a tiny incision in the back. Small tubes called dilators are used with increasing diameter to enlarge a tunnel to the vertebra.

A portion of the bone is removed to expose the nerve root and disc. The surgeon uses either an endoscope or a microscope to remove the ruptured disc. This technique causes less muscle injury than a traditional discectomy.

Identify the Cause

First, understand that outside of cases of trauma a herniated disc does not occur overnight. It may seem like you "threw your back out" all at once, yet it was a process of weakening over time that allowed your disc to suddenly become noticeably problematic.

Many people have a herniated disc without pain. It's only when the bulging disc or inner material from a herniated disc press against a nerve that pain results.

Discs are primarily composed of water. As we become older (after the age of 30), the water content decreases, so the discs begin to shrink and lose their shape. When the disc becomes smaller the space between the vertebrae decreases and become narrower. Also, as the disc loses water content the disc itself becomes less flexible.

While aging, excess weight, improper lifting and the decrease in water in the discs all contribute to the breaking down of discs, the primary cause of a herniation or bulge is uneven compression and torsion that's placed on the discs.

This uneven pressure is caused by imbalances in muscles that pull the spine out of its normal position. This forces your body to function with what I call a physical dysfunction. Every human being develops these dysfunctions over time and eventually they cause enough damage to create pain if left uncorrected.

The first step to recovery is identifying the dysfunctions you have and the muscle imbalances which created them. We have found that there are four primary dysfunctions that are either directly responsible for, or contribute to, nearly every single case of back pain or sciatica.

If you've never heard of muscle imbalances before it may not be your doctor's fault. Sadly, most healthcare professionals have never been taught the basic human anatomical and biomechanical approach used for identifying muscle imbalances. Once you've identified your dysfunctions and imbalances, then it's time for step two.

Treat the Symptoms

You can't correct the problem if your pain is so severe you can't move. So in this step you'll implement various strategies to help reduce and manage your pain so you can focus on correcting the dysfunction(s) that are responsible for your pain.

The jelly centers of your spinal discs are roughly 70% water. Gravity squeezes water out of these discs throughout the day as you go about your regular activities. That's how you can lose as much as ½ of an inch in height by the end of the day. Perhaps you've noticed as you re-adjust your rear view mirror before driving home from work. It's also this thinning of your spinal discs that might lead to more pain late in the day.

While you sleep most of this fluid gets soaked back into your discs. But if you're dehydrated or don't get enough sleep your spinal discs aren't able to fully recover. So one of the easiest things you can do as you start treating a herniated disc - or even to help avoid one - is to drink plenty of water (not soda, coffee, etc.) and regularly get a good night's sleep.

Many people turn to medicine, especially non-steroidal anti- inflammatory drugs (NSAIDs) like ibuprofen and naproxen at the first sign of pain. While inflammation almost certainly plays a role in your pain, there are significant health risks in taking them.

A better strategy is to cut back on inflammatory foods such as sugar, dairy, fried or processed foods. Introduce more fresh fruits and vegetables into your diet. And again, water should be your beverage of choice when working through pain.

You can also supplement with proteolytic systemic enzymes which actively reduce inflammation throughout your body and help your body recover from injury. While systemic enzymes won't directly cure a herniated disc, they will help reduce inflammation easing pain and making recovery much easier.

When pain flares up, a local topical ointment can offer quick pain relief. Our favorite is Rub-On-Relief which combines the all-natural pain reliever Arnica proven as powerful as prescription anti-inflammatories with MSM, menthol and other powerful ingredients for fast pain relief and actual healing power.

Finally, and we've truly saved the best symptom treatment for last when it comes to herniated discs, is spinal decompression. The reason it works so well is it relieves the pressure your vertebrae place on your spinal discs.

This reduced pressure gives a herniated disc room to return back to its normal position. Sometimes a herniated disc will suddenly recover from spinal decompression alone.

Another excellent device for decompression of the lower and middle spine is the Nubax® Trio. This device is incredibly easy to use and can provide even more decompression force than an inversion table, though it won't help herniated discs in the upper spine and neck.

Treat the Cause and Condition

Herniated discs are primarily caused by uneven pressure. Think of driving a car that's out of alignment. The tires wear unevenly due to more pressure on one edge than the other. Keep driving without fixing **the problem and sooner or later** you'll **experience a blowout on the worn side.**

The effect of postural dysfunctions on spinal discs is similar. Uneven pressure caused by muscle imbalances cause the less-pressured side of the disc to bulge or rupture, squirting the jellylike interior through the fibrous disc membrane into the spinal column. Picture stomping one end of a jelly donut - the jelly would be pushed out the other side.

Even if a treatment like spinal decompression helps you, if you don't take care of the problem that caused your disc to rupture it's just like replacing that blown out tire while leaving your car's alignment uncorrected.

That means getting lasting pain relief requires correcting the postural dysfunctions that are putting pressure on your discs. Correcting those dysfunctions requires eliminating the muscle imbalances that caused them.

Specific stretches to relax the overly tight muscles combined with targeted exercise of weak stretched out muscles restores the natural balance of tension between them. Once that balance is restored the muscles will maintain your spine in proper alignment allowing your herniated disc to heal - and stay healed.

Lumbar Traction for the Relief of Lower Back Pain and Sciatica

The benefits of lumbar traction for the relief of lower back pain and sciatica have been well known for years. Physical therapists and chiropractors utilize lumbar traction with long-term results all the time for their lower back pain and sciatica patients.

Chiropractic and physical therapy clinics may often time refer to this form of treatment as spinal decompression. The procedure can be done manually with the help of your healthcare professional or mechanically via a special traction table.

It may also be done quite effectively by you! Manually, you can use various techniques to distract your own lower lumbar spine and get relief of lower back pain or sciatica symptoms.

The purpose of this guide is to provide for instruction on how to perform seven different self-traction techniques that can be accomplished in the comfort of your own home with very little to no monetary expense.

The seven techniques listed towards the end of this e-Book are done so in no particular order.

It is recommended you try each of them whenever possible, and make a determination for yourself as to their effectiveness.

Spend the most time on those self-traction techniques that seem to be the most beneficial, give the most relief, and seem the easiest to perform.

What is Lumbar Traction?

There are two types of traction, static or constant and intermittent.

Static traction is the kind used years ago in hospitals. A small force was applied for several hours or days to a patient lying down in a bed.

This is ineffective at getting separation of spinal structures necessary for the relief of sciatica pain or lower back pain symptoms.

Intermittent traction is a forced applied alternately and released at different intervals. Since this is more easily tolerated, greater forces can be used.

There are three modes of application:

1. Manual: This is done through position and handling of a force applied by yourself or someone else. The amount of force cannot be accurately determined.
2. Mechanical: This type of traction is done via equipment available at a hospital or clinic. Since the equipment applies the force, usually some kind of indicator measuring the amount of force is used.
3. Positional: Through the use of position, a sustained force on the lumbar spinal column can be obtained.

The techniques used here in this guide are mainly manual (you apply the force) and positional.

Each of these modes can be extremely effective and I personally use technique #1 quite often in my clinic for treatment of sciatica. In fact, I do not even own a mechanical traction machine.

When is Lumbar Traction Used for Back Pain?

You may want to check with your physician before attempting any kind of lumbar spinal traction.

I will list the most common reasons (indications) and most common reasons NOT (contraindications) to use lumbar traction. These are non-negotiable. As your condition falls into the contraindicated list, do not perform these self traction techniques. Your condition can be made worse.

At all times, use common sense and stop anytime you feel extra pain or discomfort. If you are not sure, stop performing the traction technique and seek professional assistance for your condition.

These techniques would probably work better as they are used in conjunction with professional help, then instead of professional help alone. Thus, hastening your recovery time and reducing the amount of time needed with your healthcare professional. This saves you both time and money!

The Correct Treatment of Herniated Discs

When experiencing back problems or herniated discs the first person to contact is a neurosurgeon or orthopedic specialist, who may then obtain a further opinion from a neurological specialist (neurologist), especially if the pain is no longer limited to the back alone.

The nature of the complaint determines the therapy

Treatment of a herniated disc depends on the symptoms. First priority is always the so called conservative therapy, which consists of active (e.g. physiotherapy) and passive (e.g. heat treatment, massages) treatment methods – supported by pain relieving medication, if required. An attempt with acupuncture, relaxation therapy, spinal training or medical strengthening therapy. However, should none of these Methods help, surgery may be considered.

Conservative relief: therapeutical precision work

Non-surgical therapy targets the precise and gentle development of muscles, reléase of tension and relief of pain. Physiotherapeutic exercises and medical strengthening therapies are particularly suitable for targeted muscle development.

Massages loosen tense muscles. Stretching treatments to relieve the strain on the disc are also helpful, and pain-relieving and anti-inflammatory medication also support therapy. Doctors sometimes administer these drugs not only in tablet form, but can alternatively infuse the active ingredients directly where needed (infiltration procedure).

The operation: a good chance for severe cases

There is no doubt about it: nobody likes to go under the knife. However, for many patients with herniated discs, surgery is the only chance of permanently getting rid of their complaints and finding a way back to their original quality of life. Conservative procedures such as physiotherapy are often no longer sufficient, especially if the surrounding nerves are already affected and the pain has become unbearable or even crippling.

During the course of this operation, the surgeon removes the protruding disc tissue pressing on the nerves.

Exercise Guide for Lower Back Pain

One of the core messages for people suffering with lower back pain is to REMAIN ACTIVE. This leaflet will help to guide youthrough various exercises, activities and positions which can help to alleviate or to avoid lower back pain.

Positions Which Ease Acute Lower Back Pain

Remember to breathe deeply and regularly whilst stretching and exercising, this will help you to oxygenate the body, eliminate carbón dioxide and to relax fully.

a) Lie on your back, bend your legs and slowly pull your knees up to your chest, breathing out as you pull in:

b) When lying on your back in bed, bend your knees and place a cushion under your calves:

c) When lying on your side, place a cushion under your upper leg and arm:

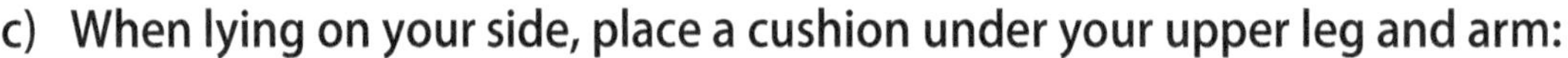

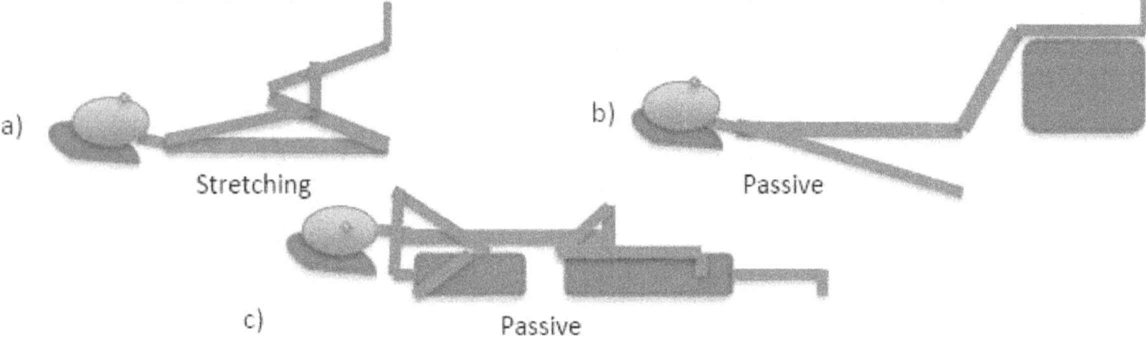

How to Manage and Prevent Lower Back Pain

The pelvic tilt is crucial and must be fully mastered before attempting any lower back exercises. It not only helps to ease lower back pain but also strengthens the support

<u>muscles around the lower back and abdominals and is vital in maintaining the spine in its correct position.</u>

A) Pelvic tilt Position 1:

Lie on your back with your knees bent, your feet flat on the floor. Relax your abdomen and inhale through your nose, then press your lower back into the floor, exhaling through your mouth tightening your abdominal muscles andpressing your lower back into the floor.

Hold this position for a few seconds, relax and start again:

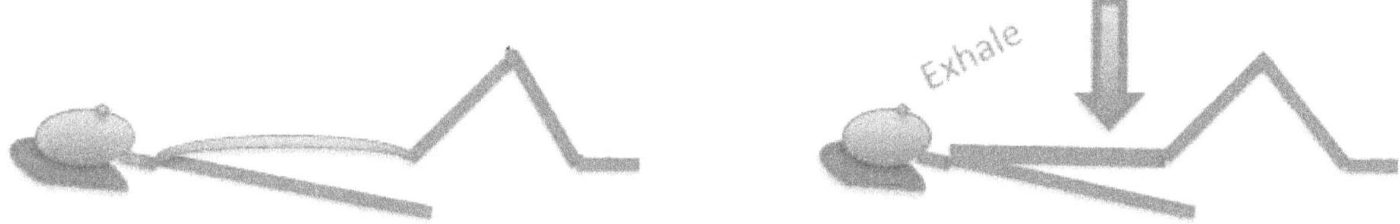

b) Pelvic tilt Position 2:

Stand and lean back against a wall with your legs slightly bent and your feet forwards, away from the wall. Inhale and then exhale as you tighten your buttocks and abdominal muscles and press your lower back into the wall. Your shoulders and head should be relaxed. Hold this position for a few seconds, relax and start again.

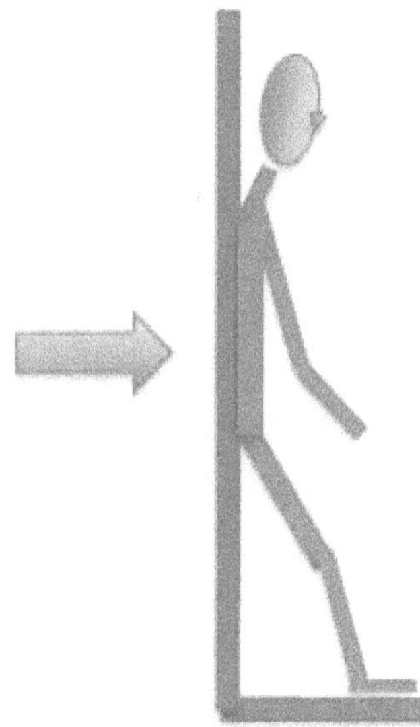

d) Once you have mastered the pelvic tilt, you should be able to do it when simply standing (legs slightly apart and bent):

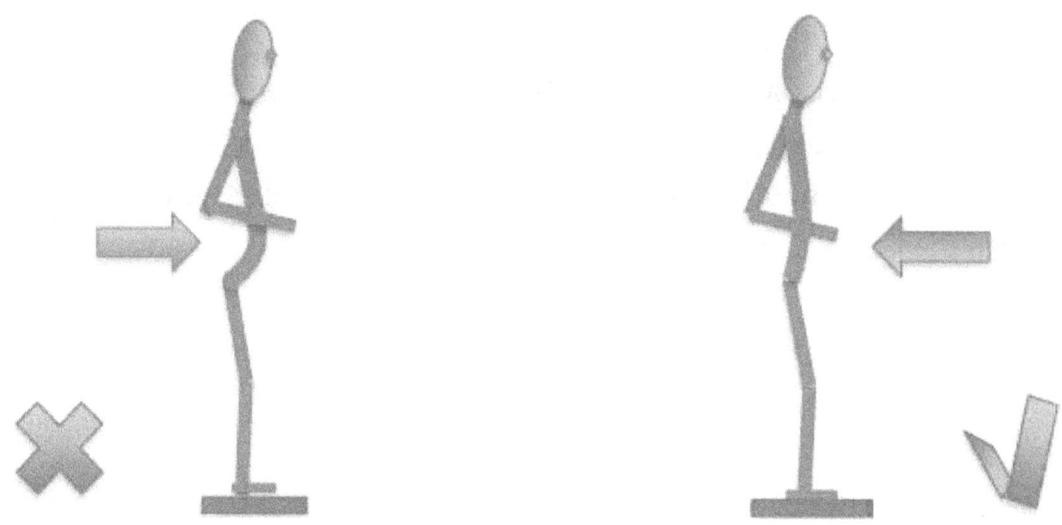

Stretching and Exercises

If you have a herniated disk or other disk problem, please contact your health care provider before attempting these exercises. If you are experiencing an acute attack of lumbar pain, wait until it has eased before attempting the exercises.

Exercises that stretch and strengthen the muscles of your abdomen, spine and legs will help you maintain a good posture and to keep your spine in its correct position.

To be effective, the exercises need to be carried out REGULARLY (10mins every day) and TENACIOUSLY (over several months at least). Movements should be smooth and measured with no jarring, they should NOT provoke pain.

a) Hamstring Stretch

Lie on your back and repeat the pelvic tilt as seen in step 2a), ensuring that your lower back is pressed into the floor. Place your left leg down with knee slightly bent. Hold your right thigh in both hands so that your knee is pointing to the ceiling. Straighten your right leg. You should feel a stretch at the back of your thigh (hamstring). Hold a moment and repeat with your left leg.

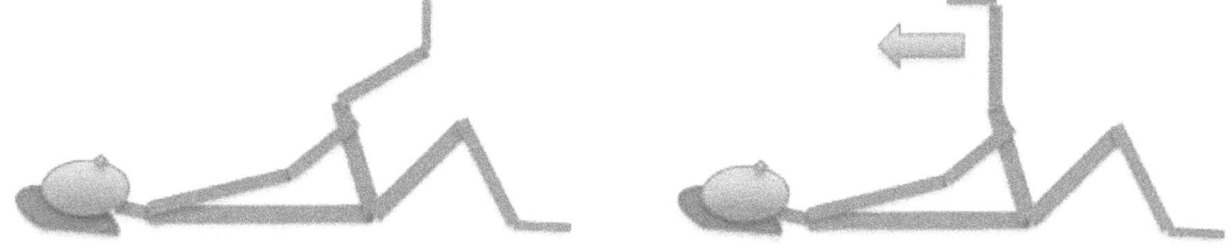

b) Cat Stretch

Get on your hands and knees (hands below shoulders and knees below hips), let your head drop down and then arch your back up as high as it will go. Hold the position then repeat several times. Make sure you keep you back flat when you release the position, do not let your back sag.

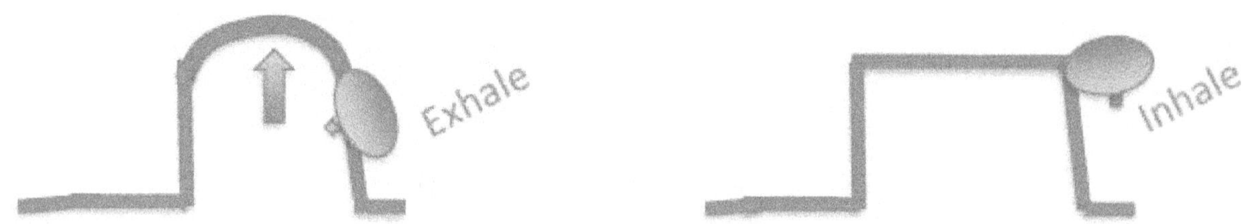

c) Partial Curl Exercise

This exercise helps to strengthen the central abdominal muscles. Lie on your back with your legs bent and resting on a chair. Tighten your abdominal muscles and press your lower back into the ground. Keeping your chin off your chest and with your hands stretched out in front of you, curl your upper body forward until your shoulders clear the floor. Exhale as you come up. Hold then relax down. Repeat 10 times. Build to 3 sets of 10

d) Partial Twist Exercise

This exercise helps to strengthen the waist muscles. Begin as with exercise c) but instead of keeping your arms outstretched, place your hands behind your head and lift one shoulder blade off the ground at a timewithoutpulling on the neck. Exhale as you come up. Hold then relax down. Repeat 10 times on each side. Build to 3 sets of 10.

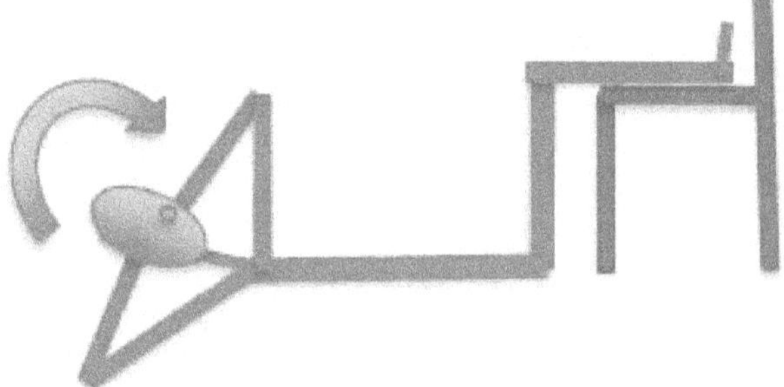

e) Dorsal Muscles Exercise

Lie on your front. Tighten your buttocks and abdominal muscles. Slowly lift one leg off the floor by a few centimetres, keeping your leg straight. At the same time lift the opposite arm by a few centimetres. Hold and slowly lower both limbs. Repeat with the opposite leg/arm. Do 3 sets of 10.

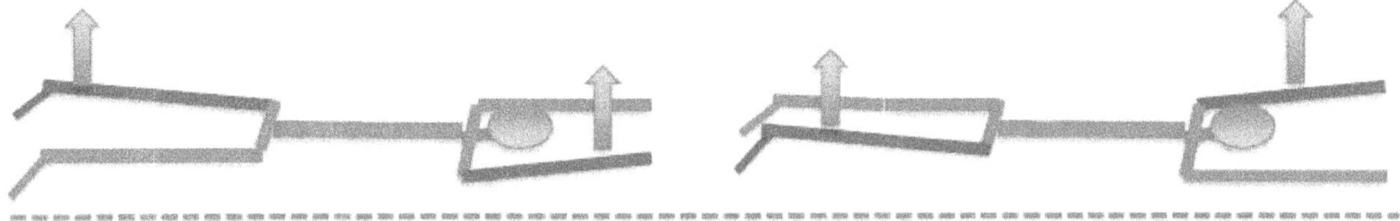

Regularly Stop and Stretch Throughout the Day, Even When at Work

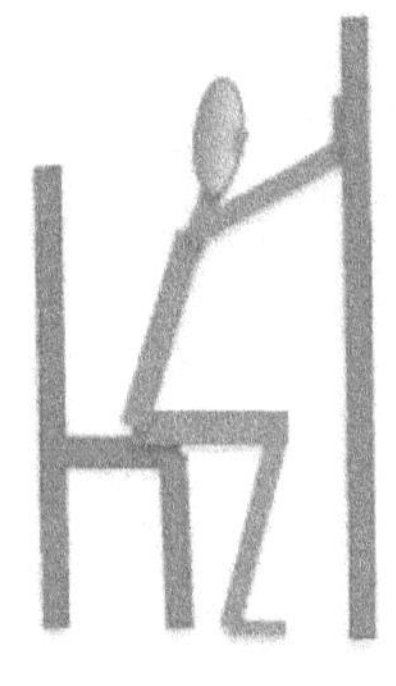

1)
Sit a foot away from the wall, with your arms stretched up and your hands against the wall.

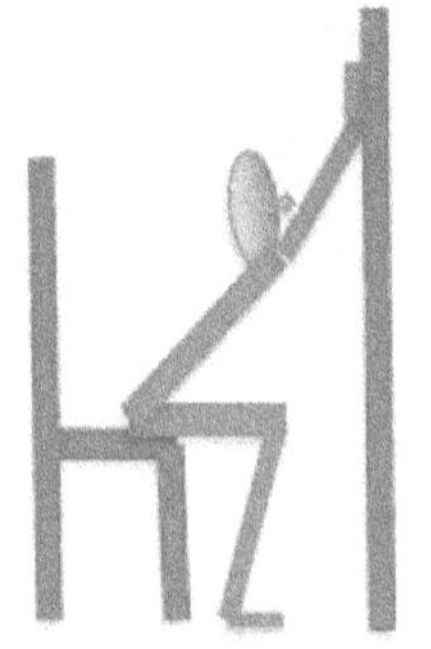

2)
Press your upper body forward and down, look up. Repeat 10 x

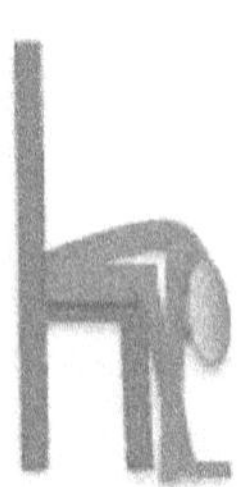

Let yourself fall forwards, head between the knees, arms hanging down. Hold 1 to 2 min. then slowly roll back up, one vertebrae at a time.

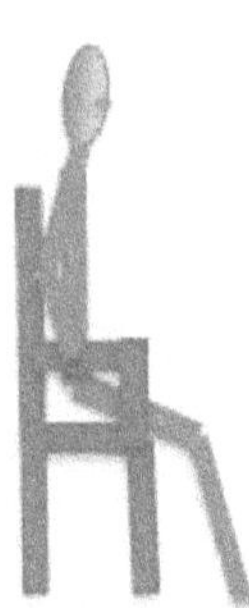

Push up from the armrests with both arms and allow your lower body to relax, feeling your back stretching out.

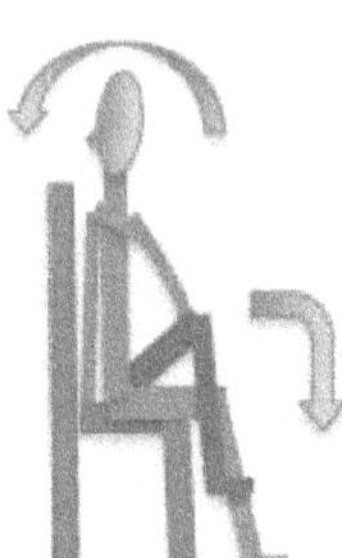

Cross your left leg over your right. Keeping your back straight, place your right hand on your left knee, the other hand behind your back and twist. Hold, then repeat in the opposite direction.

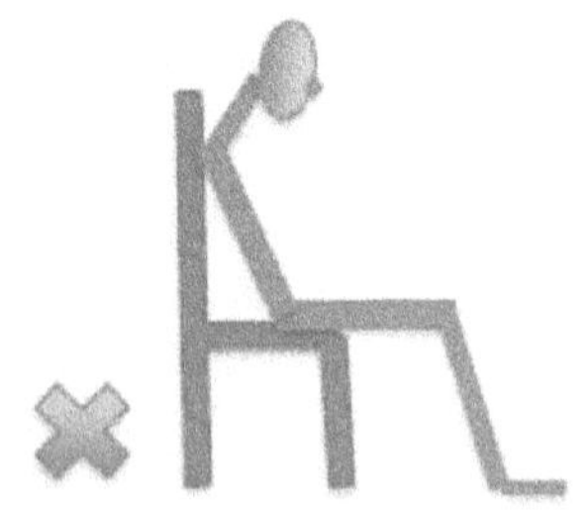

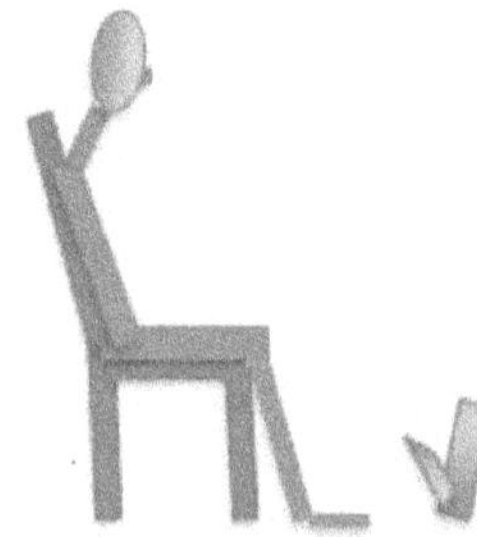

Sit with your buttocks against the back of the chair to ensure correct lumbar support. Both feet should be placed firmly on the ground.

POSTURE WHIST LIFTING:

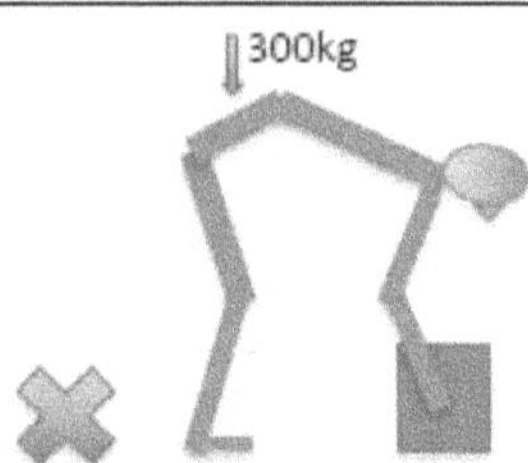

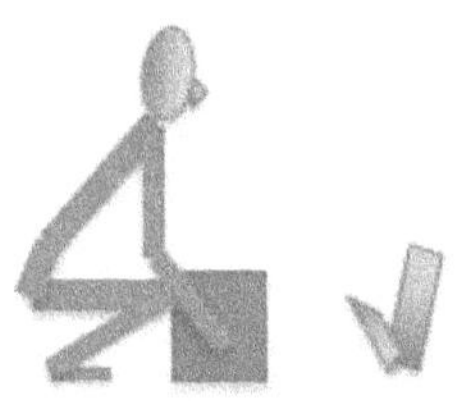

Bend your legs to pick up an object. Never lean forwards

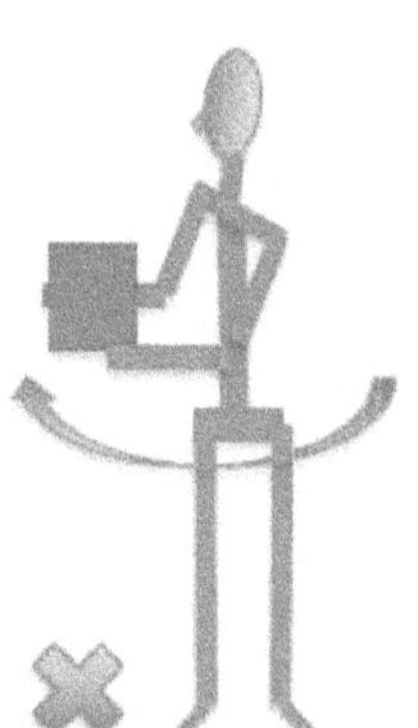

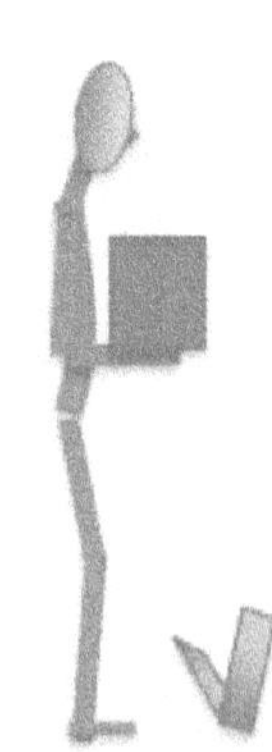

Hold the load close to your body. Never turn and lift at the same time.

Lumbar Self Traction Techniques

Technique #1

This technique is also known as positional distraction because it looks to separate the involved segment by way of position and gravity alone.

Super Important Fact: You must lay the non-painful side over the pillow (so if you have sciatica down the right leg, you would lay on your left side).

Let us say you have sciatica down the right leg. You must lie on your left side with a firm pillow rolled up about 12 inches in diameter under the top of your hip. Place a pillow between your knees.

Keep your knees slightly bent and allow your upper shoulder to roll back slightly. Lie in this position for a maximum of 15 minutes. Once you time is done, go directly onto your stomach for two minutes before getting up.

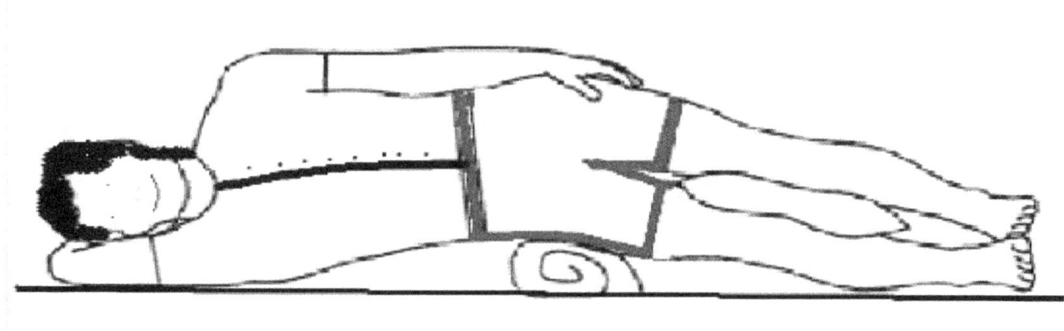

Technique #2

Lie on the floor with your lower legs supported on a chair or sofa. Hips and knees should be at 90 degrees.

Gently push against your thighs with both hands. Hold this for 2 minutes. Repeat 5 times.

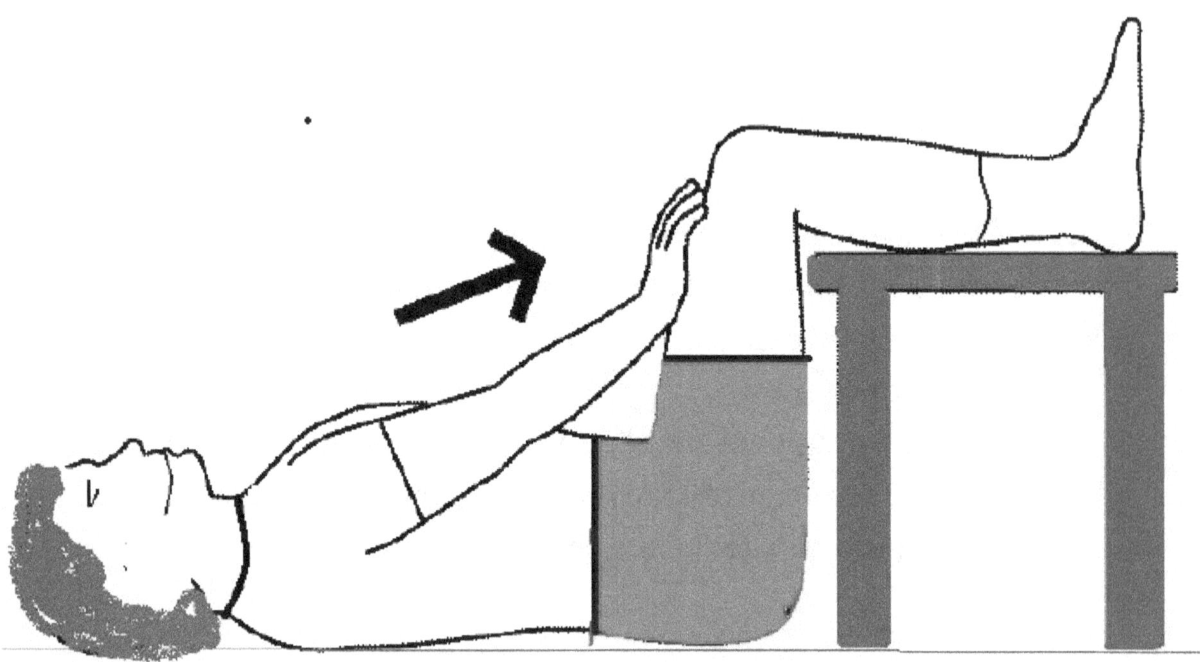

Technique #3

Lie in front of a doorway on your back with your knees bent and with bare skin touching the floor to provide friction. Raise both arms overhead and hold a cane or broom against the opposite side of the doorway. Gently pull with your arms against the cane. Hold this for 2 to 3 minutes. Repeat 5 times.

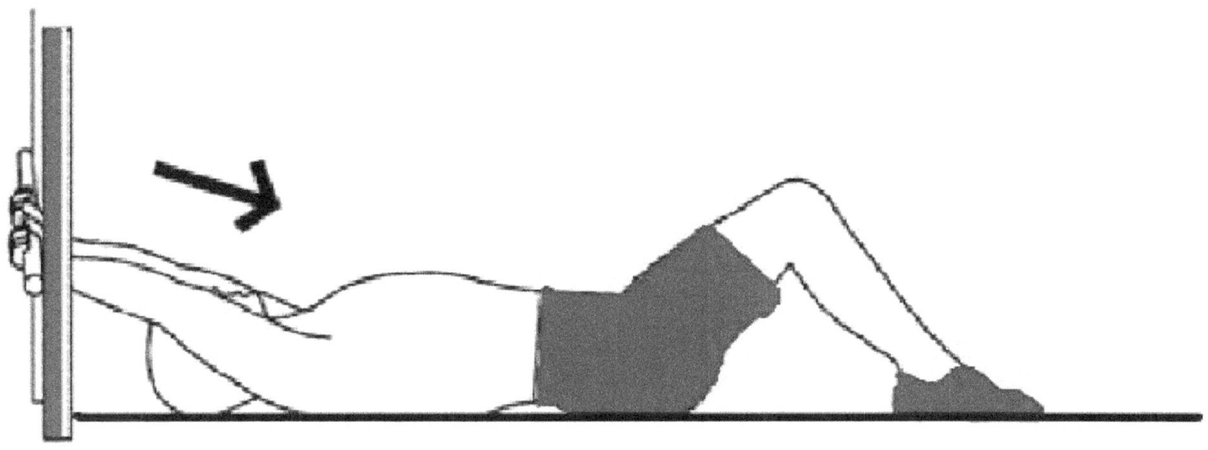

Technique #4

Lie flat on the floor in the center of a doorway with bare skin touching the floor to provide some friction. Hold a cane or broomstick in front of you across the doorway. Push against the cane with both arms. Hold this for 2 to 3 minutes. Repeat 5 times.

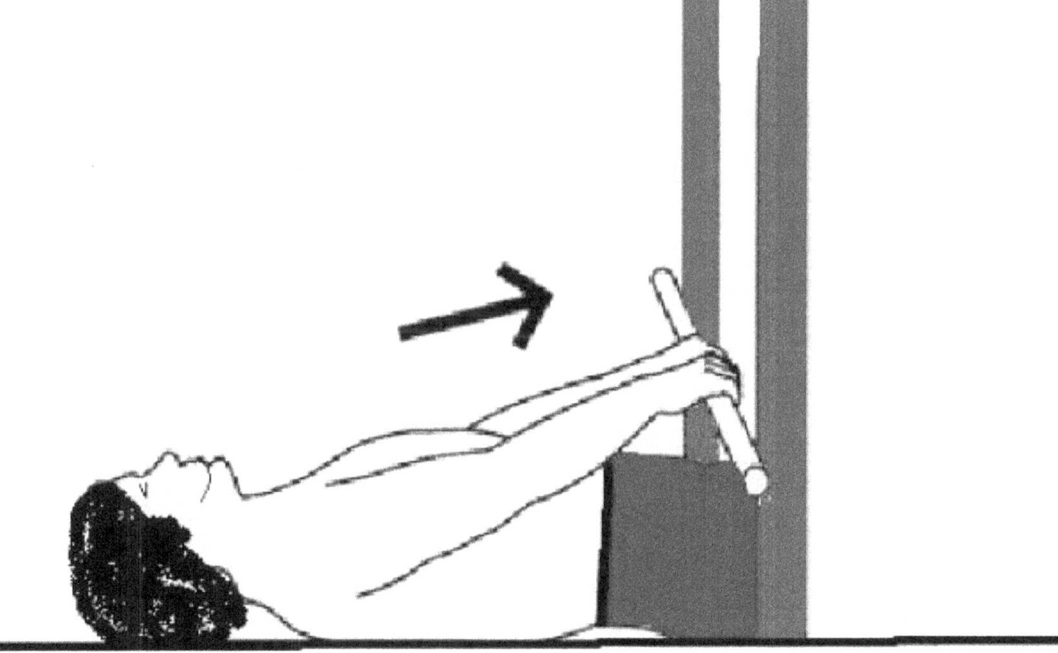

Technique #5

Lie on a firm mattress with your head at the edge of the bed. Bend your knees and raise your arms overhead so you can grasp the edge of the mattress. Try to keep your trunk relaxed as you gently pull by just bending your wrists. Hold this for 2 to 3 minutes. Repeat 5 times.

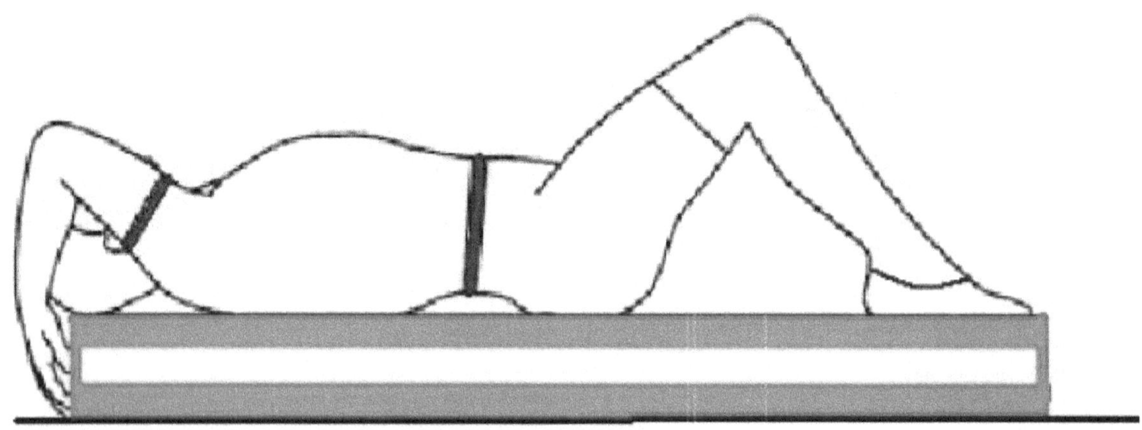

Technique #6

Sit on the edge of a firm chair with hands holding the seat of the chair on both sides. Slide your buttocks off the edge of the chair and relax your body while supporting yourself with your arms. Hold this position for a maximum of five minutes. Perform twice daily as possible.

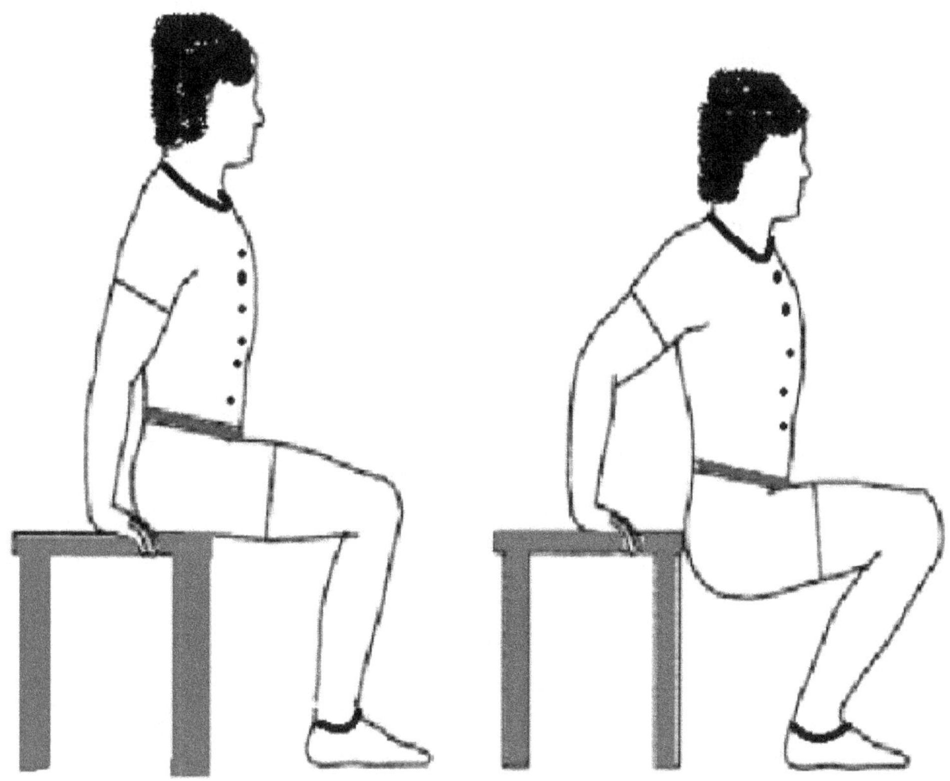

Technique #7

Hang from a chinning bar. Some door frames may have ledges thick enough to grasp and sturdy enough to support your weight. Relax your back and legs. Maintain this position of elongation for as long as you can and do not to exceed 10 minutes.

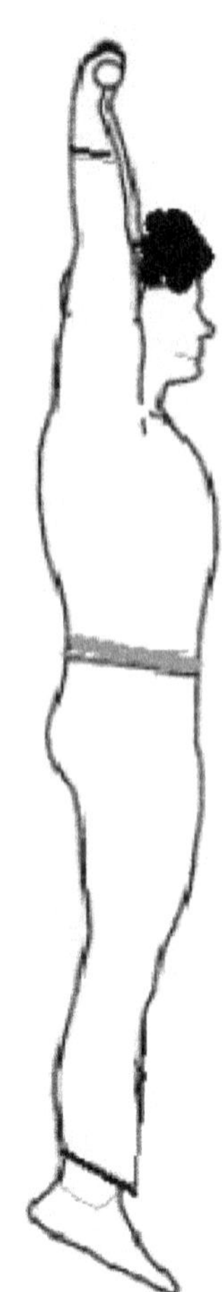

By Edgar Ortega M.